THE INSIDER'S GUIDE TO LOSING WEIGHT AND KEEPING IT OFF

THE INSIDER'S GUIDE TO LOSING WEIGHT AND KEEPING IT OFF

Vipin Marwah

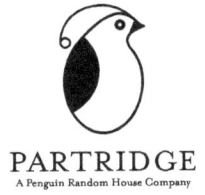

PARTRIDGE

A Penguin Random House Company

To order additional copies of this book, contact
Partridge India
000 800 10062 62
orders.india@partridgepublishing.com

www.partridgepublishing.com/india

Contents

Preface

If you are among those people who weigh more than they should, this book is for you. If you have tried to reduce weight once or many times but did not succeed, this book is for you. If you have succeeded in losing weight but have not been able to maintain it, this book is for you.

This book will present the science and art of weight loss, in easy to understand terms. Once you understand the underlying concepts, you will understand the reasons behind over-eating and food cravings. Reading this book will take you more or less the time it takes to watch a movie, and hopefully it will change your life.

After reading this book you will be able to enjoy food with taste and nourishment like never before. You will start to enjoy food without guilt or fear of getting fat. You will be healthier, happier and you will lose weight.

Moreover, after following the principles taught in this book you will have increased energy levels through the day. You will sleep better through the night. Your blood sugar levels and blood pressure levels will improve for the better and you will decrease your risk of developing diabetes, hypertension and other lifestyle diseases in the long run.

I have experienced the weight loss journey myself. Despite being a wellness professional and fitness practitioner for years, even I gained weight. I looked up conventional literature again and again during my quest for weight loss. All I found was advice on avoiding fats like the plague, eating 5 to 6 meals a day, smaller meals at night and doing "cardio" based workouts (aerobic exercise) along with strength training. I was following most of it but still slowly gaining weight, and I could not understand why. Also, lethargy and gastrointestinal discomfort had become a part of life. And what of the grogginess, getting up in the morning wasn't complete until the first cup of coffee hit the lips. Graying and hair loss were the icing on the cake. Are you experiencing any of the above? Yes, I have been there too.

Weight loss is easy! There is very little that you need to do in order to lose weight. You just need to know to do the right things. With the right knowledge and understanding you can bring about the right kind of changes in your body weight.

Your lifestyle defines you and also your weight. Empower yourself with the right knowledge and use it to create a brand new you. You will be amazed to see how easy and pleasing the process is. You will come through improved, in this case 'change is not just good, it is better'.

Chapter 1

The rise of obesity and the opportunities in weight loss

More than six billion humans, 10 times that number of animals, add to that birds, insects, trees, plants, bacteria, fungus and other living organisms total up to somewhat close to infinity. Trillions of things are happening on the planet right now. The world is changing every second, as you read along; life, is evolving. Every species is working to become more adept at surviving and thriving. Among all this hustle-bustle there are scores of people who are waking up to the idea of changing for a healthier lifestyle. Congratulations! You are one of them.

We all naturally want our bodies to look and feel good. Being overweight creates a sense of imperfection within us due to this natural inclination. When we make efforts and lose weight, looking at the mirror every morning is very uplifting and motivating. Weight loss improves self-esteem improves life.

Besides looking and feeling good, we are also constantly bombarded with information about the health benefits of weight loss. At times, we make half-hearted attempts to make it happen. And sometimes, we make highly enthusiastic but very short-lived attempts to change our lifestyle habits. The net outcome is that even with the desire and knowledge of health benefits, a lot of us are not able to generate enough momentum to obtain and maintain meaningful and sustainable weight loss.

Why you haven't been able to lose weight?

In my career working in the wellness industry, I have met thousands of people who have taken to regular exercise and or dieting and became fitter, but have not lost weight. Sometimes they have even gained weight after starting an exercise regimen. Even more often some of them have lost weight temporarily, but gained it back just as quickly.

The solution to a problem is something that actually solves the problem. When weight gain is the problem, solutions are often just theoretical. To lose weight, according to popular science, you must eat non-fat food, frequent mini meals through the day, and small meals at night, consume copious amounts of fiber, count calories, exercise regularly and control your appetite with a conscious effort. If you have ever attempted all this, you might have experienced either of two outcomes. Either you were not able to do all of it at the same time, or, even if you maintain all this discipline for a few days, it didn't last long.

This prescription to win the battle of the bulge seems akin to advising someone who is drowning in water, to hold his breath. If you don't breath you will surely not drown, but you cannot 'not-breath'. And then we conclude, 'Oh! He drowned because he had no control over his breathing'.

A solution would be something that can actually be done. If the commonly accepted panacea to obesity described above was actually working, we would not have an obesity epidemic today. Is there a way to stop this? Good news! It is possible for an overweight person to find his path to a leaner body.

The rise of obesity

Our minds can sense change only when it is quick, but we can't really see this obesity epidemic since it has been slowly spreading over the last few decades. When we do attempt a guess at why it is so, we blame mechanization and automation, along with human weakness aka laziness and gluttony, for these seem like obvious reasons.

What we fail to notice is how come we do not eat lesser now that we work less? Doesn't the human body have a mechanism to control how much we eat so that we fulfil our requirements, no less and no more? (just like all wild animals, none of whom are obese) Research does point to a hormone called 'leptin'. This hormone regulates appetite. Abnormality in the working of this hormone in the body makes us eat more than we should. Question is, why has this abnormality set in among such a large proportion of human population (and human population only) in the last few decades?

When something effects a large portion of an entire civilization, it takes a long patient look at its history to understand what went wrong. Unfortunately, mainstream scientific research has taken a symptomatic approach and is treating the symptom without attending to the cause. The real reason lies in how with mechanization and automation we have not changed the pattern of food production and consumption. Unlike animals, we don't eat whatever grows nearby. Neither do we hunt down our meat for consumption. We live in a complex interdependent socio-economic environment, where availability of food is a function of price, storability, transportability and packaging convenience.

Grains and starches are sources of quick energy, they have become even faster acting energy sources due to food processing. This kind of a diet would make sense to a largely manual labor driven civilization, not to the advanced industrial-techno-cyber-automated society that we have become. If majority of us were working in farms and handicraft, we could keep eating this quick energy stuff and burning simultaneously through an entire day's manual labor. Those days are gone, but we continue to consume them because economies of scale and food processing facilitates cheap, mass production of mountains of turbo charged energy boosting 'soft foods'.

Why you should lose weight?

Weight gain comes with a fairly large portfolio of health risks:

Cardiovascular disease
Diabetes
Hypertension
Osteoarthritis

Stroke
Depression
Asthma
Fatty liver
Cirrhosis of the liver

The likelihood of acquiring one or more of these diseases increases as you gain weight. And I am sure that most people have heard these things. Would you want to lose weight because of the fear of these? Even more important question, "Can" you lose weight because of the fear of the above diseases? Sorry, but fear does not make you lose weight.

The assumption underlying this fear motivation, which is widely available and sometimes as free advice, is that the overweight person is deliberately eating away to obesity by choice. Next time anyone points a finger at you to say "Don't you care about yourself, getting fat eating all day?" Please reply back, "I eat because I get hungry, not because I want to get sick. So, back off."

Help is here. First thing you have to appreciate is that you don't get hungry by choice, so it is not your fault. Do not feel guilty!! Second, you will very soon be learning why this uncontrollable appetite exists and how to stop it without having to take a single pill, starvation, procedure or exercise.

The opportunities in weight loss - The positive approach

There is always a positive side to everything. If you are overweight right now, you can avail the following benefits by losing weight:

Become heart healthy
Improved brain function
Improved sleep
Improved energy and vitality
Improved psychosocial outlook
Improved fertility
Improved mobility and pain free joints
Improved blood glucose control
Improved blood pressure
Lowered cholesterol and triglycerides
Regain your drive for physical activity

All these amount to deceleration of the aging process.

Investing in health

Health is a value and a very intrinsic one indeed. You have 'one' body which has all those organs, bones, muscles and other tissue. The body has many subsystems that work together to create one integrated system for normal functioning. Whatever extra weight you put on and carry around puts extra work load on all of those subsystems and compromise normal functioning. By getting rid of extra weight and keeping it off, not only will you live longer, but your quality of life will improve.

Good news - Weight loss will make you exercise ready

It is commonly believed that lack of exercise makes you fat, although it has only a marginal effect on your tendency to gain weight. That's why reversing the situation will only have a marginal effect, if at all. Now look at the problem from the other direction.

Becoming fat renders you unable to exercise or play sport. Being overweight puts excessive strain on our system. Any sensible organism will instinctively protect itself against physical activity when it is already overloaded with excess body weight. As we gain weight, our drive to exert diminishes. First we stop taking interest in any physical activity that does not come from necessity, like playing sports or running or gym-ing. With time and as weight gain epitomizes it also interferes with our drive to indulge in physical activity that is necessary like daily chores and work related movement.

Losing that excess weight is the path to finding the joy of voluntarily testing your physical limits in sport. As you lose weight you will find renewed motivation and ability to become physically active. Once again, do not chastise yourself for not exercising, it is not your fault. First you will lose weight and then you will 'want' to exercise.

Lifestyle change

What you will learn from this book is a lifestyle decision and choice. It is not a diet plan that you have to follow for a limited period of time in order to lose weight temporarily.

Adopt it as your lifestyle to always maintain your natural weight, avoid lifestyle diseases and remain healthy.

Your body is your home and the vehicle of life, nourishing it, purifying it, unburdening it, easing it and pleasing it is your primary karma. Treat it like you would treat an invaluable magic lamp, it is the only one you have and it is capable of miracles.

Your health is priceless, for it can't be bought or sold. The moment you decide that you value your health, making the right lifestyle choices becomes a rewarding experience. Take that decision right now and the rest will fall into place. The only words you need to say to yourself are "I am ready to change".

Chapter 2

Goal setting

This is where your journey towards weight loss begins. The power of goals is unparalleled. Whatever you want from life becomes concrete when you give it the words, numbers and visualization of a goal.

Goals = Numbers + Words + Visualization

It is easy to generate the words and numbers that comprise your goal. However the third component: visualization is a much more dynamic process and often neglected.

Why are goals important?

Goals give our desires and aspirations a concrete form that becomes an image in our mind. It makes it easier for you to stay connected with your target and develop determination for achieving it. The more you think about your goal, the more you will work towards achieving it. In fact, your subconscious mind then points you towards any and all opportunities present in your environment that would move you further towards your goal.

How to setup goals?

Numbers:

Dates — An open goal can turn into a far-fetched dream unless we put a time line on it. Put a fixed date by which you will have achieved your goal.

Specific number - We live in a world of quantified performance. Most goals will have a quantifiable dimension, whether money or square feet or kilograms or percentage. Specific numbers make your goal a fixed entity and give you a particular number to chase, for example, if your goal is to save a million bucks for your child's education, you won't stop until you've reached a million. Imagine setting goal that said, "I want to save a lot of money for my child's education". It's very ambiguous and has no specific quantification.

Words:

Present tense — Your goals have to be in the present tense, meaning that you have already achieved the goal. Eg: If your goal is to become the Senior vice president of your company, the words should be "I am the Senior Vice President of my company"

Positivity — Words should be positive. Do not include words about what you don't want. Eg: If you want to change your job, the words should be "I am now creating a new job opportunity for myself" (the words should not be "I don't want to be in my current job" or "I don't like my current job so I will get a new job")

Visualization:

Visualization is the magical component of goal setting. It adds the magic of emotional energy to your words. We all do visualize from time to time; consciously and sometimes unconsciously. For example, when you imagine proposing marriage to your partner, you think of every detail of where and how you would do it. Or when you enter a competition, you imagine how you would react when you win.

Harnessing the power of visualization to achieving goals is a key to success. It is nothing but, taking yourself on a mental and emotional sojourn of having already achieved your goal. Preferably, in a quiet place, with eyes closed, you imagine how you would feel after having achieved your goal. What all you would do, who would you share your success with, what will you say to yourself and to others, what will be the rewards you will reap for your success, how you would walk, talk and feel and the list is endless. You can imagine yourself in endless situations, the idea is to live that feeling of having achieved your goal. When you recognize your own emotions linked to your goals, they make you an unstoppable force. These emotions become a driving force when you practice them on a daily basis. They easily replace any feelings of doubt or fear that might challenge you during your journey.

Here is how to apply the process of goal setting in case of weight loss.

How to check your weight?

- Buy your own weighing scale, and buy a good one.
- Check your weight at the same time of day, once every week.
- Remove shoes and accessories before checking weight.
- Maintain a log with date and time, either on computer or in a diary.

How much weight do you need to lose?

Following is the BMI (Body Mass Index) table that gives the range of weight you should be in i.e. Ideal weight basis your height:

MALE			FEMALE		
Height in Feet	Height in Meters	Ideal Weight	Height in Feet	Height in Meters	Ideal Weight
4' 6"	1.3524	28 - 35 Kg	4' 6"	1.3524	28 - 35 Kg
4' 7"	1.3778	30 - 39 Kg.	4' 7"	1.3778	30 - 37 Kg.
4' 8"	1.4032	33 - 40 Kg.	4' 8"	1.4032	32 - 40 Kg.
4' 9"	1.4286	35 - 44 Kg.	4' 9"	1.4286	35 - 42 Kg.
4' 10"	1.454	38 - 46 Kg.	4' 10"	1.454	36 - 45 Kg.
4' 11"	1.4794	40 - 50 Kg.	4' 11"	1.4794	39 - 47 Kg.
5' 0"	1.5	43 - 53 Kg.	5' 0"	1.5	40 - 50 Kg
5' 1"	1.5254	45 - 55 Kg.	5' 1"	1.5254	43 - 52 Kg.
5' 2"	1.5508	48 - 59 Kg.	5' 2"	1.5508	45 - 55 Kg.
5' 3"	1.5762	50 - 61 Kg.	5' 3"	1.5762	47 - 57 Kg.
5' 4"	1.6016	53 - 65 Kg.	5' 4"	1.6016	49 - 60 Kg.
5' 5"	1.627	55 - 68 Kg.	5' 5"	1.627	51 - 62 Kg.
5' 6"	1.6524	58 - 70 Kg.	5' 6"	1.6524	53 - 65 Kg.
5' 7"	1.6778	60 - 74 Kg.	5' 7"	1.6778	55 - 67 Kg.
5' 8"	1.7032	63 - 76 Kg.	5' 8"	1.7032	57 - 70 Kg.
5' 9"	1.7286	65 - 80 Kg.	5' 9"	1.7286	59 - 72 Kg.
5' 10"	1.754	67 - 83 Kg.	5' 10"	1.754	61 - 75 Kg.
5' 11"	1.7794	70 - 85 Kg.	5' 11"	1.7794	63 - 77 Kg.
6' 0"	1.8	72 - 89 Kg.	6' 0"	1.8	65 - 80 Kg.

Source: http://doctorsdunia.in/files/2010/03/BMI_Chart1.png

If you are outside the maximum range of weight in your height category, there is room for weight loss. However, there are exceptions like pregnancy, extreme muscle mass, water retention or obesity due to medical conditions and heavy bone frame etc. In these cases weight loss might not be an option.

You can choose your target anywhere in the normal range, it does not have to necessarily be the lowest possible weight. In case you are grossly above the maximum weight in the range, you might want to choose to goal for the highest figure in your range. For example, you are a female at 5'6" and your weight is 85, which is grossly above the maximum in your range (65Kg) ie. 30% above maximum. You might want to goal for 65 kg. Losing 30% of your weight would be quite an accomplishment, you can always re-goal to a lower weight once you reach this goal.

Numbers:

Dates – By when do you want to target reaching your target weight? It is all right to lose on average around 5% of bodyweight per month. In the initial month you might lose more than this, but the average would stay in this range. How quickly you lose weight is dependent upon how insulin resistant you are as of now. (insulin resistance has been explained later)

Example – Today is 1st of Jan., you are a 5 ft. 8 inch tall male weighing 90 Kg. Your goal weight is 70 Kg. You are looking at shedding 20 kgs.

5% of starting weight (90) = 4.5 Kg

Time required to lose 20 kg @ 4.5 Kg per month = 4.4 months (20/4.5)

You can reach your target weight by 12th of April.

So you have your numbers ready:

Goal weight – 70 Kg
Date of achievement – 12/4/2014

Words:

Present tense – We always state our goal in present tense because we want to feel victorious every time we say the words. We say them every day as a part of our visualization.

Positive – We use positive words and avoid words that point towards anything that we do not want from life.

"Today is 12/4/2014 and I weigh 70kgs, I feel light, happy and healthy".

Visualization:

The magic of visualization multiplies with practice.

When to visualize?

It is a great idea to visualize early morning because your mind is fresh and it is a great way to start your day with positive feelings.

However, the rule with visualization is that the more you do it, the more powerful it becomes. Also, remember that whenever we are faced with a challenge or merely negative thoughts about failure, we start visualizing that as well. We think of ourselves as having failed and then put ourselves down with all kinds of imagined negative things: I can't change, I am destined to be overweight, life is not fair, I will never try to lose weight again, I hate thin people etc. All this is also visualization and it affects us negatively.

So the prescription is: Do your weight loss visualization once early morning and as many times as possible throughout the day. Specifically do it more number of times than the number of times negative thoughts of failure come to your mind.

What to visualize?

- A calendar that shows the date of goal achievement.
- You looking thin, wearing your favorite clothes and feeling light.
- Feeling happy to be at a healthy weight.
- Sharing your accomplishment with your friends and family.
- Meeting people or doing things you were earlier shy of doing because of your weight.

The list is endless, you could visualize just about anything that you would want to in your new avatar. This is your mind, it is the inception point of where your real world is created. If you've been there in the mind, you will go there in the body.

Key element: emotional energy

How did the visualization make you feel? The objective is to be able to generate the emotional experience. When happy and exultant emotions are experienced it raises your spirit. It is like a switch that generates motivational electricity inside you. Keep practicing and it will become your attitude.

This is a power inside you that can change your life. Mostly, people experience emotions as a result of what happens around them. Few realize that you can generate the right emotions with the power of your mind. Use it! miracles will begin to happen.

Chapter 3

WHY?
(Science of obesity)

Imagine a car, now imagine driving to the fuel station and getting a full tank. Once full; your car will use all the fuel and you will need to get more once the gauge drops to the 'empty' sign. That's normal. The key thing here is that this car will not need any more gas, till the entire tank full you put in is used up. Now imagine another car, imagine going to the fuel station and getting a full tank. You start driving and after a few kilometers the cars 'low fuel' warning signal starts blinking and then you come to a halt even though the fuel gauge shows there is still fuel left in the tank. The fuel is there but your car refuses to use it and just halts. You add some fuel to the already existing inventory and the car starts working again. That would be abnormal, isn't it? There has got to be something wrong either with this car 'or' the fuel that you put in.

If you have excess weight, your body is kind of behaving like the second car you imagined. You eat energy rich food and your body should use all of it before you start feeling hungry again. Instead you actually feel hungry every couple of hours even though you haven't used up the energy you consumed from the last meal. That is abnormal, isn't it? Hunger is an unpleasant sensation that only eating can dismiss, hence you eat. Result is that stores of unused energy are just sitting under your skin in the form of fat. There has got to be something wrong with either your body 'or' the food that you are eating. Wouldn't it be worthwhile to find out where the problem is?

In order to find out the answer to this puzzle, you will need to understand a few simple things. You will need to understand the term 'glycemic index'. Sounds fancy, but it is not very difficult to grasp.

Glycemic index – stands for the rate at which any given food releases energy into the body on being consumed, in comparison to other foods. The higher the rate at which energy is released into the body on being consumed, the higher the glycemic index rating is.

For example - Table sugar is the fastest releaser of energy among all food and hence has a glycemic index value of 100, which is the highest value.

So it very simple, faster the release of energy, higher the glycemic index rating.

We will refer to Glycemic Index as 'GI' from here on.

GI = Glycemic Index

How does it matter whether energy is released fast or slow into the body by any food?

Let's go back to the example of the car. Just like a car needs the right mix of fuel and air to function properly, which is why there is a carburetor, your body also needs energy at a rate that it can handle. Too much fuel released at one go and the car's carburetor gets flooded, the engine does not start and you see lot of smoke coming out of the tail pipe. Similarly, if the food that you eat releases too much energy at a rate faster than your body can handle, it creates problems.

When food is consumed it goes to the stomach, where it is processed so that energy is released into the blood. When too much energy is released too fast, it raises blood sugar. High blood sugar is toxic (which is why diabetics are given medicines that control blood sugar).

Under normal circumstances when food is consumed, glucose or sugar is released into the blood. The body (through pancreas) then releases insulin which in turn captures energy or sugar from the blood and gives it to muscles and organs for use and some to fat deposits for later use. Insulin is a hormone and regulates storage and delivery of energy and other nutrients.

However, when a food with high glycemic index value is consumed, too much sugar is released into the blood and consequently too much insulin is released to remove sugar from blood. The job of insulin is to remove excessive sugar from circulation. When there is excessive sugar and insulin in circulation it converts too much energy into fat and stores it away. Muscles can only store a limited amount of sugar as glycogen for immediate use. Hence all excessive sugar in blood gets stored as fat.

As energy is removed from blood circulation and stored as fat blood sugar levels go down. Excess insulin still in circulation; then clears your blood of all sugar. As a result blood sugar level drops below normal which further makes you feel lethargic, sleepy and hungry again.

To summarise, the problem with energy being released too fast by foods with high glycemic index value is that it promotes fat storage and makes you too hungry too often:

Step 1 - It raises blood sugar levels too high and too fast.

Step 2 - It triggers excessive insulin release to bring sugar levels down.

Step 3 - Insulin extracts sugar from blood and stores it away as fat instead of being used.

Step 4 - As almost all of blood sugar gets stored as fat, energy levels drop below normal.

Step 5 - You start feeling hungry again.

Step 6 - You again consume high glycemic index value foods and go back to step 1.

This vicious cycle goes on and you keep eating, keep storing fat and keep gaining weight.

What effect does glycemic index value have on appetite?

High glycemic index value food increases appetite. The fat storage process is triggered due to insulin secretion, which is caused by excessive blood sugar. When all blood sugar gets stored away as fat, there is no readily available source of energy left for the body. This results in feeling low energy, sleepiness and hunger.

How do foods with 'low' glycemic index value release energy? How does that effect appetite?

Foods with low glycemic index value release energy at a slower rate. Due to this slow release, blood sugar levels remain within normal or tolerable range. As a result of this sustained slow release, there is no trigger of excessive insulin release and hence only minimal storage of energy as fat. This also means that blood sugar levels do not drop below normal. Hence, you do not feel hungry after eating. So the consumption of low glycemic index value foods will reduce your appetite as compared against high glycemic index foods.

Going back to the question: Whether something is wrong with the body or the food that we eat? Why do we feel hungry even though the energy from the last meal consumed is still not utilized?

The answer is simple: Something is wrong with the food that we eat. Because we consume too much of high glycemic index value foods, we keep getting hungry while energy from the previous meal gets stored as fat.

How valid are these scientific principles?

In the last 100 years many have researched, written and propagated about the effect of glycemic index on fat storage. Dr. Atkins among the most popular. Gary Taubes has written a comprehensive book that covers the science behind obesity and low carbohydrate lifestyle, "Why we get fat? (and what to do about it)".

There is a significantly large and growing scientific community that supports these scientific principles. Because of their efforts millions of people around the world have lost weight and maintaining it through a low carb lifestyle, its time you also changed your lifestyle.

Chapter 4

WHAT?
(Science of losing weight)

The reason for becoming overweight is consuming excessive quantities of high GI value foods. So obviously by reducing or eliminating this consumption we can stop gaining weight. However, our objective is to not only stop gaining more weight but also lose the excess weight that we already have. Here is how.

Going back to the example of a car, if you found out that the fuel in your car is not appropriate, you will surely source the right type of fuel and start using that. However, what about the fuel that is already sitting in your car and refuses to burn, you will need to figure out a process for removing it. You could have the tank removed and the fuel emptied, but that would need a mechanic and would be expensive. Or another solution: you could use a different kind of fuel that would not only stop further storage of fuel as dead weight but also make the existing dead weight fuel burn off, over a period of time. The second choice is much easier and doesn't require any mechanical procedure.

In the case of your own body, your goal is to remove the excessive deposits of fat around your body. You could go to a surgeon and ask for a liposuction prescription, but that would be expensive, require bed rest and comes with all the risks of undergoing surgery. Or you could start eating the right type of food which would not only stop further storage of fat, but also burn off existing body fat. The second option is easier, cheaper and doesn't entail any risks.

This is what you need to do:

Eat the right mix of foods, which translates into a lower GI value and stabilizes your blood sugar levels. It not only stops storage of excessive energy as fat but also, helps the body to derive energy from existing fat stores. With limited insulin release and its complete utilization for delivering energy, your body doesn't stay in storage mode. As a result, you don't feel lethargic due to lack of energy and you don't feel hungry very frequently.

Do all foods have a GI value?

No.

How to distinguish between foods that have a significant GI value from the others?

Food is made up of three macronutrients or major components:

Carbohydrates – Mainly provide energy – Directly impact blood sugar – Have higher GI value than other macronutrients.

Proteins – Mainly provide growth, repair and maintenance of the body – Do not impact blood sugar adversely – Have significantly lower GI value than other macronutrients.

Fats – Mainly provide energy, growth and development and – Do not impact blood sugar adversely – Have negligible or no GI value.

Almost all food that you consume has varying quantities of all the three macronutrients. The more carbohydrates a food has the higher the impact on blood sugar, especially if it is high GI type.

Protein and fat have very little impact on blood sugar. Hence, any food that has a significant amount of protein or fat with little or no carbohydrate will have no GI value.

Which are the foods that we consume in large quantities and also have high glycemic index value?

This list explains why obesity is so widespread. These are foods that comprise more than 50% of daily consumption for most people. Some of these are consumed during every meal and are considered to be staple foods. These are the primary reason for making you overweight. Following is the list:

- Roti (wheat)
- Parantha
- Bread (white and brown)
- Rice
- Pasta

- Macroni
- Noodles
- Sugar
- Potato
- Naan (Maida)
- Aerated cold drinks
- Packaged chips, corn puffs, rice puffs etc.
- Biscuits and cookies
- Patties
- Samosas
- Breakfast cereal
- Idli

The list is not exhaustive but covers the most commonly used foods in the Indian context.

The objective:

Eat less or don't eat foods with high glycemic index value and eat more foods with low glycemic index value or no GI value. Remember, by doing this you will stabilize your blood sugar, hence not feel too hungry and overfeed and hence you will lose weight.

Is it that simple to lose weight?

It almost is, however, there is a hurdle that might challenge some of you: Insulin Resistance.

What is insulin resistance?

Insulin resistance develops because of extended periods of overconsumption of high GI foods. Every day for years, sometimes a lifetime; a lot of people over consume these foods. This leads to release of too much insulin every day and throughout the day. With time, among a lot of people, the body stops partially or completely responding to insulin.

Remember, the job of insulin is to store away energy as fat. Insulin resistance is the phenomena whereby some or all of your body's cells reject insulin and block the storage of energy through its action, because of years of abuse, leaving sugar in the blood. However, sensing high levels of blood glucose, the insulin release mechanism ie. your pancreas; still overloads the system even further. Unfortunately the pancreas cannot sense that there is already insulin flowing through the body.

During the time it takes insulin to find the cells that are receptive to it, sugar remains high and more insulin is dumped into the system. Over flooding takes place till sugar levels go below normal. But by this time your pancreas has released so much that there is still more than necessary insulin in your blood. End result is that your system stays in fat storage mode even after removing all sugar from blood. Within an hour of eating, you eat that snack with your tea or coffee and there is already insulin waiting to store it away. In all probability the snack you eat is a cookie or some other starch laden high GI edible which again furthers the flood of insulin. The vicious cycle continues.

What happens to us because of insulin resistance?

Insulin resistance is the pre-diabetic stage. After years of insulin flooding, among a lot of people, either the body completely stops accepting insulin that is produced or the pancreas gives up and produces very little or no insulin at all. The resulting stage is what is known as diabetes.

How does insulin resistance effect your ability to lose weight even with low GI dietary lifestyle?

Depending upon how insulin resistant you are right now, it will make it difficult for you to lose weight even after reducing the consumption of high GI food. This happens because even little bit of high GI food and also low GI food would trigger release of insulin, and because it is not efficiently used by your cells to allow removal of blood sugar, the pancreas will over release insulin and hence you stay in fat storage mode. Which means that whatever other food you consume will also keep getting stored as fat and no energy will be available for normal functioning, making you hungry.

We will touch upon insulin resistance again at a later stage. Let's go on to understanding more about what needs to be done in order to lose weight.

Which foods to eat, if not the ones mentioned above in list? (After all, they are a big percentage of the average Indian meals)

There are some carbohydrate rich foods that have a low glycemic index value and can be consumed. However, you would need to consume more of fats and proteins in order to get enough energy to cater to your requirements.

Say that again, is this book suggesting that people should eat more fat? Isn't fat the enemy?

Yes, you are being asked to eat more fat. The reason why you became overweight is not eating too much fat in your diet. You have been eating too much high GI carbohydrate, which is making you fat. Hence you need to remove or reduce the carbohydrate to lose the extra weight. Fats are energy rich and will do the job 'without putting your body into fat storage mode'.

Won't eating fat also add weight?

No it won't.

Why won't eating fat make you fat?

Because high fat foods do not have any effect on your blood glucose. Hence they do not promote secretion of insulin. Your body will stay in energy burning mode. The fat you eat will be used for energy throughout the day.

Won't the fat in food get stored as fat?

No, it will not get stored as fat but only under the condition that you do not consume High GI foods. This dietary fat will be digested and circulated in your body as 'fatty acids'. Your muscles, brain, nervous system and other tissue will use them by converting these fatty acids into fuel.

How will the body break down dietary fat into readily usable energy instead of storing it as fat?

When you do not consume High GI value foods for an extended period of time, your body changes gears. And in this new gear, the liver starts producing 'ketone bodies'. Ketone bodies are molecules that are produced by synthesis of the fatty acids. They are then circulated through blood and are easily used as energy by the body. In essence, you will train your body to start using fat for energy.

Why hasn't this been told to you by your doctor or other people?

As I mentioned earlier many books have been written about this in the last hundred years. However, mainstream science is still slow in accepting this scientific principle of nutrition. The Indian nutritional advisory still recommends the same high carbohydrate and low fat dietary approach which has been around for forty years. Obesity has spread to epidemic proportions during this period. In very simple words, the advice we have been getting, is wrong

Conventional medicine still resists the idea of eating high fat high protein diet. However, change is the way of life and slowly things are changing. There is enough scientific evidence to back up weight loss through low carb, high fat and high protein dietary lifestyle. There are hundreds of thousands of people around the world who have adopted this lifestyle and have lost weight permanently. And also successfully avoiding lifestyle diseases like diabetes, hypertension and heart disease.

As a country, Sweden is leading this new change. They have already accepted this as the norm and their national health advisory recommends low carbohydrate and high fat diet.

Which foods have a low glycemic index rating?

- Lentils
- Bengal gram / chic peas
- Most vegetables
- Peanuts
- Beans
- Flour made from lentils (Besan)

Which foods are high in good fat and / or protein?

- Ghee
- Olive oil
- Butter
- Cheese
- Cottage cheese
- Cream
- Red meat
- Chicken
- Eggs
- Fish
- Nuts: Almonds, cashew and walnut
- Tofu

Nutrition is not complete without vitamins

Vitamins do the job of catalysts, helping the breakdown of food into nutrition for the body. With population explosion agriculture has developed technologically, but it has put too much pressure on land as far as productivity is concerned. The use of pesticides and germicides along with absence of crop rotation has resulted in adverse effects on the nutritional value of food produced. The result is that food has lesser nutritional value especially vitamins and minerals.

Deprivation of vitamins also results in malnutrition, which means that even though a lot of people eat too much, they are still malnourished. So, taking vitamin supplements is a good idea to complement your new dietary lifestyle. There are many over the counter multi-vitamins that can do the job for you.

Chapter 5

HOW
(how to go through the change process?)

It is clear what needs to be done in order to lose weight. The next step then is to understand how to do it.

Basically you can choose either of two alternative strategies:

1. Eat less of high GI foods or eliminate them - while adding to your consumption of "fat and protein".
2. Eat less of high GI foods or eliminate them - while adding on your consumption of "low GI foods".

Following are some principles you need to follow as a permanent lifestyle in both the strategies:

A simple way to success is through the use of this acronym: '**LOWGI**'

Leave sugar out of your life.
Omit packaged snacks
Weigh fruits, not more than 100gm/day
Govern your High GI food intake
Indulge yourself, eat to your fill

Leave sugar out of your life.

Sugar enters the body and within few seconds it finds its way into the blood stream, makes you feel energized instantly. The human body is not designed to handle this kind of surge in blood sugar. It really floods the system with insulin which then starts packing off everything as fat only to make you feel sapped of energy within few minutes.

All beverages, snacks, packaged food and fast food contains sugar in some form or the other. It is the highest GI value food that is available out there. Treat it like you would treat poison. There are sugar substitutes available and their long-term effects are dubious. Within the scope of this book, without going into too much detail, sugar substitutes are not recommended.

It is challenging to leave sugar because it fancies your taste buds. The damage it does far outweighs the momentary pleasure of taste it generates. It takes a few days to get used to living without it, but as you get past the craving, you will begin to appreciate the taste of things you would otherwise not have without sugar. You will feel much better about your health.

Omit packaged snacks

Packaged snacks like chips, puffs, cookies, muffins, chocolates, sweets etc. all contain varying quantities of high fructose corn syrup, starch, added sugars, potatoes or rice. Particularly high fructose corn syrup is a very common ingredient in most packaged snacks. These are all high GI value foods. They give instant relief to your hunger pang but just as quickly make you hungry again within a few minutes. You consume them, not because they are nutritious but because they are:

- Very easily available and
- Come in attractive packaging
- And mouthwatering flavors.

These characteristics make them an easy buy to your slightest temptation.

Weigh fruits, not more than 100gm/day

Fruits are a special category, they don't raise your blood sugar like sugar does. Yet, they contribute to fat storage all the same through the liver. All 'fructose', that's the name of the sugar in fruits, gets converted to fat in the liver. Further it gets broken down into usable energy as and when your body is not in storage mode. Have fruits in moderation, if at all. Approximately 100 gm per day is more than enough. If you are someone who is really finding it hard to lose weight, it would be a good idea to just completely avoid fruits for a month.

Govern your high GI food intake

Glycemic index values of foods are of key importance. Most of the common culprits are easy to remember ie. White flour, sugar, cereals, potatoes and rice. You should keep a printed list of high GI value foods handy. You could take a copy of Page 33-34 and keep a folded copy in your pocket.

When you are faced with a situation where you can't figure out the glycemic index value of food that you are about to eat, either read the label or ask the cook/vendor: 'what are the major ingredients?' Then refer to the printed list to see if the major ingredients belong to the High GI list.

In time you will memorize the commonly consumed and easily available high GI foods.

Indulge yourself, don't starve

One of the most important factors that effects changing your lifestyle is not having to starve. Starvation is an unpleasant feeling and humans don't like it. The good news is that you do not need to even try resisting food when you feel hungry in this new lifestyle.

Just eat to your fill, only eat the right kind of foods. When you avoid high GI foods you are creating an environment inside your body that will promote sustained release of energy through the day. When insulin release is lowered, so is your hunger, since you will maintain optimum level of sugar in circulation for the body to use for energy.

Hence, over a period of time your hunger pangs will reduce on this kind of nutrition.

Besides these principles you must learn to listen to your body in order to develop more control over how you feel through the day:

Learn to listen to your body.

Feeling sleepy after food

A very usual signal that your body gives you is feeling sleepy after your meals. This is a very common phenomena, people feel very sleepy after having their lunch. Think about it, you have just consumed energy rich food, instead of feeling energized you feel drowsy, why? The reason is high GI value food. Your sugar levels peak due to high GI food intake and excessive insulin is released. Insulin stores away all available sugar in blood as fat. And you end up feeling drowsy and sapped of all energy.

Learn to listen – When you do feel this way after food, review the ingredients of your meal. If you find that you ate too much of the high GI stuff, try to reduce them in your next meal and see whether you still feel sleepy few minutes after food. Slowly you will be able to control this reaction from your body too. By having more of low GI foods or fats and proteins rather that high GI foods you will not feel sleepy because the energy supply will be regularized. Rather than peaking at the time of eating and then subsequently dropping to very low levels, your energy levels will be normal for a longer time after you eat and hence not make you feel drowsy.

Eating without hunger

Eating too many times can become addictive for some people. Eating again and again through the day can create a psychological dependence wherein you eat food or snacks even when you are not hungry, but simply out of habit or as a means of taking a break.

Learn to listen – When you are about to eat randomly, check whether you felt the urge to eat or are you just doing it to kill time or just to break out of routine. There are other ways to take a break, like drinking water or lemonade (without sugar of course) or just do some stretching or call a friend to chit chat.

Strategy 1

Eliminate high GI foods - while adding to your consumption of "fat and protein".

- It's simple and easy to follow.
- It will give better and faster results.
- Even if you are insulin resistant it will work.
- You completely avoid all high GI value carbohydrate foods.
- Eat unlimited amounts of fats and proteins.
- Eat very little of low GI value foods.

List: High fat and protein rich foods you can eat:

Ghee
Butter
Animal fats
Olive oil
Nuts: Peanuts, walnuts, almonds and cashews
Fish
Red Meat

Cream

Cheese

Chicken

Bacon

Cottage cheese (paneer)

Eggs

Strategy 2

Eat less of high GI foods or eliminate them - while adding on your consumption of "low GI foods".

- If you are insulin resistant, results will be slow and not as good as the first strategy.
- Elimination of high GI foods is more effective than reducing them.
- Your diet should have a lot of protein.
- Whatever low GI foods you choose to consume, should be minimal. It is difficult to say how much is ok to have. Since it depends upon how insulin resistant you already are.
- Do not starve yourself, eat to your fill. Starvation will lead to failure in keeping away from high GI stuff.
- This strategy is difficult to monitor and apply since it requires calorie counting.

Who would choose this strategy and why?

This strategy for losing weight by controlling high GI foods can be chosen by those who are weary of eating too much fat, because they have learnt all their life that eating fat is bad for health.

List: Low GI foods you can eat

Lentils, pulses and legumes
Chic peas or Bengal gram
Roti made from pure bengal gram flour
Peanuts
Green leafy vegetables
All vegetables except potatoes, pumpkins and parsnips
Whole milk
Skimmed milk
Peas
Beans

In summary, this strategy simply implies that in your current standard Indian meal plan, the only thing you need to change is to:

Decrease or eliminate the quantity of roti, bread, rice, sugar and potato (or any variation of these like parantha or naan).

AND

Increase the quantity of the other things that you eat along with these. Like vegetables, pulses, curd, salad etc..

Answers to specific questions that you might have when you start following the simple glycemic index principle:

How much of roti, bread, rice etc. is ok to consume?

Since the goal is to lose weight, it requires reduction in the quantity of high GI value foods. So the answer is simple, whatever quantity of roti, bread and other high GI value foods you consume as of now, it should be reduced to as low as possible. For example if you consume 4 rotis reduce it to 3 or 2. Once you get used to it, you can reduce it further to 1 and even zero.

Wont it lead to starvation ie. eating so much lesser?

It won't because you don't need to eat lesser.

How will reducing these foods not mean eating lesser and feeling starved?

You will not feel starved because you must increase the quantity of low GI value foods in your meal. Most of the high GI value foods are consumed with other foods and not on their own. For example roti, bread and rice are not consumed standalone but rather with vegetables, pulses, chicken, fish and other gravy cuisine. A lot of times they are also accompanied by salads and curd.

Simply increase the quantity of these other foods ie. Veggies, chicken and curries etc, such that you get your fill. Which means while reducing the quantity of roti, rice etc. Eat extra portions of chicken, veggies, pulses, curd and other low GI foods.

How much extra quantity of low GI foods can be consumed?

You were earlier eating without any conscious control over quantity. Continue to do the same. Which means, eat till you feel satiated. Only, because now you will be eating a better mix of high and low GI value foods, you will not end up feeling hungry as quickly as you used to. Remember it is not about reducing consumption, rather it is about balancing your GI mix so that your blood sugar does not yo-yo through the day.

What you should and what you should not eat?

Depending on availability and accessibility you can learn to eat the right mix of high and low GI value food. If everything that is available to you is high GI value then you have to eat very little and look for something low GI at the nearest place possible.

Nuts of all kinds, peanuts are easily available and so is bengal gram. They make a good source of energy with low GI value.

Is eating foods high in fat a problem?

Eating fat is equal to eating for energy. If you compare the GI values of high fat foods with that of high carbohydrate foods, you will find that former have much lower GI ratings, sometimes negligible.

Energy from fat is released slowly, which is why eating fat is good. However, if you combine it with food that is high GI you end up storing everything as fat.

A few words on the big picture

Simplify it for yourself. Eating is something that is built into us, we would not have to learn about it from others if it were not for the controlled environment that we live in. All animals living in the wild learn to eat on their own and they pretty much maintain their normal body weight as per their species. They only use their nose and tongue to figure out what to eat. Have you ever seen an obese horse or leopard or elephant in the wild? Ever heard of a nutritionist leopard that prescribes portions to fellow leopards? Which means they have the ability to automatically regulate how much they have to eat. It's hard to believe that humans don't have such an ability. So where did we go wrong?

We, unlike animals, live in cultural, social and economic settings that force us to eat more of particular foods that are made available rather than what grows around us in natural settings. Agricultural economics, food storage and transportation costs along with marketing strategies dictate what reaches our stomach rather than our own natural preferences. Moreover, food technology advancement has empowered food manufacturers to fool our taste buds and olfactory abilities as required. Artificial flavors can make the most insipid and unhealthy food a much sought after delicacy and often an addiction.

Our body has a mechanism to tell us what should be eaten, how much and what should be avoided. Over a period of time due to sensory deconditioning we have forgotten the art of using our instincts. We end up eating whatever is widely acceptable and available. Wheat and rice are widely accepted and available because they are easiest to grow, store and transport. They have also become embedded in our culture. These factors make them the 'ideal' food to feed the masses, but, certainly not the 'healthiest'.

We can't change the world suddenly, but we sure can start with ourselves. Lifestyle diseases are as common as the common dietary lifestyle, so don't wait for an official blow to your health, it's already under threat, change starts today.

About the author

Vipin Marwah is a health psychologist and wellness consultant. He started his work in a leading hospital and laid the foundation for understanding of health related behavior among people. He has also been the General Manager of the largest health club in Delhi, India. His key skills involve connecting with people and motivating them to action their health and fitness goals. It always perplexed him to see folks who spent tireless hours working out but not losing weight in years. During his journey he experienced weight gain himself, despite following conventional advice. It was during his own quest to lose weight that he discovered how popular recommendations are not only inaccurate but are responsible for the obesity epidemic. He lost weight and has been maintaining it for many years. Now works to help others understand the science behind weight loss. Vipin has one strong message for his readers "Your body is your home, nothing in this world is worth compromising your health and well-being".